OVEREATING

Steps To Help You Stop Dieting, Binge Eating and Overcome Food Addiction Once and For All

Written by
ROBBIE GRIFFIN

Introduction

I love food. It's as simple as that. Food has always been a comfort for me. It has been there for me when things were falling apart and it has been there for me when things were wonderful. For me, my love affair with food began as a child. I remember visiting my grandfather and he would give me candy or cakes. It was his way to make you feel welcomed in his home. It was his way of showing love; and who can possibly say no to love?

As a species, humans have always linked events in our lives with food, special events, holidays, celebrations, funerals, births... Everything involves food. With food playing such a large role in our lives, why does it cause some people so much distress and not others? Why do some people know when to step away and leave food on their plates while others are incapable? What makes us overeat?

A person's love affair with food is actually a complex problem and it can cause some dangerous side effects. In this book we will discuss this very issue. We will explore various reasons as to why we overeat and the different ways to work to end the overeating problem. We will also touch on the popular fad diets and why they don't always deliver on the promises they say to lure you in. There will be a section that will help you to choose which foods to avoid and which foods to choose, both while dining out and in the grocery store. We will explain how to curb your cravings and even throw in some interesting tidbits here and there about your favorite foods—just to keep things lively!

Sit back, grab a cup of hot tea and prepare to go on a journey that will help you understand why you overeat and how you can go about ending the cycle.

Published by WOS Publishing

First Printing, 2013

ISBN-13:
978-0615935676 (WOS Publishing)

Printed in the United States of America

Table of Contents

Why Do We Over Eat?

Biology, Genetics, Emotions and Stress All Play a Role.

It is easy to assume that all overeaters are obese or overweight. It is also easy to assume it is a choice the person makes. While these statements may be partially correct, it isn't the entire truth. There are a great number of factors that go into why people overeat. For some people, it is as easy as making a choice. For other people, it can be almost a compulsion. And then for others, well, it could be a combination of both a choice and compulsion. The problem isn't as black and white as some people may lead you to believe. The grey matter often lies within your own body.

An overeater can place some blame of their overeating habits on their biology. The body is a fickle machine; and as we know, it takes maintenance and great care to keep it running well. The food you eat not only acts as fuel and gives you energy; it also gives your body a pleasurable feeling. Have you ever noticed how you feel after eating chocolates? Maybe you feel happier, more alert? This is because chocolate causes our bodies to releases hormones that will make you feel good. And like all good things, there is a line between eating a healthy amount and eating too much. By eating too much sugar, this may cause you to produce large amounts of dopamine—one of the feel good hormones.

Dopamine causes the same pleasurable feelings as when someone uses drugs to get high or climax during sex. Too much of a good thing can lead to an addiction. Addicts always look for that dopamine rush, be it with their next sexual encounter, their drug of choice, or that bite of food. Without these fixes, the addict will feel a sort of withdrawal. Their bodies crave the dopamine that they have gotten so used to. For food addicts, these cravings for food will lead to overeating and most likely weight gain.

As an associate professor at the Scripps Research Institute, in the Department of Molecular Therapeutics, Paul Kenny has suggested that overeating can also be caused by an irregularity of chemicals in a person's brain and that the act of overeating itself can change the biochemistry of the brain. Researchers conducted tests on lab rats to monitor their response to food and their reward sensors. All the rats were given the regular rat food, while one group had unlimited access to unhealthy human food and another group had restricted access to the unhealthy food. It's no surprise that the rats who had unlimited access to the unhealthy foods didn't touch the regular rat food and quickly became obese. What is surprising though, the group that had a limited time with the unhealthy food feel victim to overeating.

What this experiment shows that the less you get something, the more you are likely to over compensate when you are finally able to have it. It also shows that the obese rats with unlimited access to the bad foods had a higher threshold for feeling pleasure. This led the rats to gorge on the fatty food because they just didn't feel satisfaction that the food normally would bring.

The dopamine receptors normally found in the brain became scarce, and to get the feel good sensation the rats continued to eat and eat. This is phenomena can also be found in those of drug or alcohol addicts since there aren't many receptors, the person will over indulge in order to get that pleasure feeling.

Genetics can also play a role in the chances of someone becoming overweight, both metabolically and neurochemically. The lack of the dopamine receptors can be a genetic problem. This would explain why children of substance addicts have a higher chance of becoming an addict themselves. This can also work with food.

As with overeating, high blood sugar can be genetic. Because you are eating an abundance of "feel good, comfort" foods which are high in fats and sugars, your body can be overcome with too much glucose (sugar that is found in the foods we eat and the body uses it for energy) in your blood. This is a problem because your body can't make enough insulin to distribute and use all the excess sugar that is being ingested. Too much sugar can cause heart disease, kidney failure, blindness, and even death.

It is estimated that 75% of overeating is done because of our emotions. We often learn that food can make us feel better, even if it only lasts briefly. When we are depressed, bored, or lonely, we reach for foods that will satiate those feelings. If you're anything like me, you learned that eating food is a way to cope with difficult feelings. Someone pick on you at school, all you want is a candy bar. You had a bad day at work, you stop at any given fast food drive through and order a value meal, which is loaded with fat and salt. Just the simple act of eating can be used as a distraction from our emotions. We learn at a young age that food can make us feel happy, too. As a child you would go to the doctor for a shot, and they would give you candy to make you stop crying. If you did well on your report card, you parents may take you out to a special dinner and ice cream as a reward.

Along with our emotions being a factor in why we overeat, stress is an even larger factor. According to the American Psychological Association, 25% of Americans rate their stress levels at an 8 or above. No wonder America has an obesity epidemic. We are a very stressed out group of people! Now you may be thinking to yourself that sometimes you don't feel like eating anything when you are under stress. You are right. Stress in the short term will cause some people to lose their appetites. It is when you are under prolonged stress is when the overeating happens. It all depends on the amount of stress and how long you experience that stress, will your body produce one of two hormones.

Epinephrine is a hormone that is released most during times when you are under stress in the short term. This hormone is linked to the fight or flight response. Your body will put the need for food on hold so that you may fight or flee the cause of the stress.

Cortisol is the hormone that is released when you experience prolonged stress. Cortisol increases a person's motivation, be it for survival, fighting, participating in any kind of activity—including eating. Under most circumstances cortisol levels will become lower as the stress has been reduced, but there are instances when a person's cortisol levels can remain high if their stress response remains active.

Overeating isn't all just within your chemical make-up. It can also be engrained in you from childhood. How many times did you have to stay at the dinner table until you finished everything that was on your plate, even if you were full? We may not realize it, but by teaching your children to finish everything on their plate can stay with them into their adulthood. With portion sizes being large enough for two or three meals while eating out, it can be difficult for a person to leave food on their plates and this can cause them to over eat.

Sources for this section:

http://www.doctoroz.com/videos/tips-stop-emotional-eating

http://www.medicinenet.com/emotional_eating/article.htm

http://www.scientificamerican.com/article.cfm?id=addicted-to-fat-eating

http://www.drweil.com/drw/u/ART00524/compulsive-overeating.html

http://www.health.harvard.edu/newsletters/Harvard_Mental_Health_Letter/2012/February/why-stress-causes-people-to-overeat

What Do We Crave?

Who are the culprits and why do they plague us?

We all have them. Some people are able to avoid them and others are not. We overeaters are more likely to fall victims to the vicious 3; salt, sugar, and fats. And these are the things that we overeat. Rarely do you ever know of someone who gorges themselves on fruits and vegetables. No, these 3 are the things we reach for the most.

Sometimes the cravings can be so bad it is the only thing you can think about, but why? Why do these things taste so damn good and why do we crave them so much? In this section we will explore this. We will also delve into the world of processed foods and chain/fast food restaurants and why we crave their foods.

Salt

Sodium Chloride, popularly known as salt, is a magical substance enhances any flavor in food.

It can make vegetables taste that much better and salting meat makes it juicier and more flavorful. Not only is it a must have for cooking, it is a must have for our bodies. It is a necessary compound that our body requires to function properly. Salt (or sodium chloride) helps to regulate the balance of your fluids, relax your muscles, and it also helps your nerves transmit signals throughout the body. Without this compound you could experience mild symptoms such as headaches, nausea, vomiting, dizziness, muscle cramps, disorientation and fainting.

Although lack of salt is rare in our diets today, it can be possible especially if you have constant diarrhea or vomiting. Too little salt in the body plus the intake of large amounts of water can be very dangerous. The excess water will dilute the already low sodium in the body. This could result in some serious problems that range from seizures, coma, brain damage and even death.

Now, this doesn't mean to load up on the salt! Too much salt can be just as bad. High salt intake can result in high blood pressure which may ultimately lead to heart disease, stroke, and later death if it goes unchecked and unregulated. It is recommended that you should get between 1 and 1.5 grams of sodium and 1.5 and 2.3 grams of chloride a day.

Sugar

Often times, people are accused of having a sweet tooth. These people love sweets, be they candy, cookies, cakes; anything with sugar in it.

You would be surprised to know that sugar is in almost everything we eat. Either it is refined sugar or high fructose corn syrup. Either way you cut it, we crave it. Sugar cravings could be due to a lack of glucose in your blood (also known as hypoglycemia) or you may just need a serotonin (a chemical in your brain that makes you feel happy) boost.

Some things that may trigger your sugar cravings could be dehydration, lack of activity, stress, and sleep deprivation. These triggers are usually set off by having adrenal fatigue. The adrenal glands produce chemicals that give us energy and without glucose (sugar) the glands may not work properly. Because the body doesn't have the sugar that it needs already present in the body, you will look for in food items that will allow for quick absorption of that sugar. This boost in sugar can ultimately lead to a sugar crash, and so begins the cycle of craving sugar, getting a sugar rush, then have a sugar crash. It's a vicious cycle really.

It's best to try and regulate your sugar intake. You don't want to eat too much sugar because it could lead to diabetes. Some suggest that before you give in to the sugar cravings; try to go for a walk. Instead of sugar, your body just may be telling you that it needs to move around.

Fats

Have you ever heard the old remedy to help with a hang over? You know what I'm talking about, the one where you eat something greasy and you'll feel much better afterward? A professor of human ecology and nutritional sciences at Cornell University, David Levitsky, suggests that the craving goes back to our biology. He says that all mammals want to eat the foods that offer the most energy, fat does exactly that. Levitsky states that, "It's just that [when you're] sober, you won't usually give in to those cravings. But after a night of boozy indulgence, you lose such learned inhibitions as disciplined eating."

Hangover cures aside; we need fats in our diets. Omega-3 and Omega-6 fatty acids are necessary in our diets because they contain fat soluble vitamins A, E, and K. Not only do fats and oils provide our bodies of vitamins, they are sources of energy, they make our cell membranes stronger, and protect our nerve endings. Fats and oils also make food taste better. Ever notice how dry and bland turkey burgers can taste compared to a beef burger? Turkey is naturally a lean meat and so there aren't any fats or oils to give the meat flavor or juice; whereas the beef burgers are full of natural flavor and juice (unless it's over cooked, but that's a topic for another book).

Craving fatty foods also have emotional ties. These foods contain an amino acid called tryptophan which produces serotonin; that's the feel good chemical. This chemical can help relieve feelings of stress and anxiety and improve your happiness and well-being. Have you ever noticed the link between your emotional state and what you reach for? Let's say you had a bad day at work and you pass a local fast food place.

You know you shouldn't go there but you just crave a meal. All three of the cravings can be addressed in one high calorie fast food bag.

You've got your fatty craving from the burger and fries, the sugar craving from the soda, and the salt craving from the fries. After you eat your meal, don't you feel a little better? It's not the healthiest option, but it is convenient.

Speaking of fast food, why do we crave them? What do places like McDonalds, Burger King and the like put into their foods that make people flock to their restaurants? Affordability is certainly one factor. A person can get a meal for mere dollars if they select options from the dollar menu. The dollar menu can be an overeater's downfall, especially if you have cravings. You can satisfy your cravings and not spend a whole lot of money.

Economic factors aside, there are ingredients in fast food that can be rather addictive. I'm sure you're aware that fast food is highly processed. Fats, salt and sugars occur naturally in our food, however fast food places sell food that has been processed and pumped full of high fructose corn syrup, casein (often referred as the "nicotine of fast food"), and MSG. These ingredients combine to make food that feeds into our weaknesses for salt, sugar, and fats but yet they offer little to no nutritional value.

Salt, sugars and fats are necessary for our health. These foods occur naturally in the foods we eat and they can't be avoided. The trouble for humans, not just over eaters, is that our food is becoming so expensive it is difficult to afford food that is unprocessed. The processed foods are pumped full of preservatives, additives, hormones—it's no wonder we are overweight.

Sources for this section:

http://www.cracked.com/article_18549_8-health-foods-that-are-bad-your-health.html
http://www.shape.com/healthy-eating/diet-tips/50-seemingly-healthy-foods-are-bad-you
http://sciencemags.blogspot.com/2010/07/why-do-you-crave-sugar-salt-and-fat.html
http://www.primalpal.net/paleo-recipe-blog/63/Why-Do-I-Crave-Sugar
http://nutrition.about.com/od/askyournutritionist/f/sugarcrave.htm
http://www.webmd.com/diet/features/the-facts-about-food-cravings

http://www.fitday.com/fitness-articles/nutrition/healthy-eating/understanding-cravings-why-people-crave-fatty-foods.html

http://www.livestrong.com/article/369937-addictive-ingredients-in-fast-food

Curb Your Cravings

Some Ideas on How to Curb Your Cravings

Let's be honest, curbing your cravings isn't going to be easy. Sometimes you can get frustrated and say screw it and cave in. Don't worry, we all have a those moments. What is important is that you don't worry too much about it. Stressing over giving into your craving isn't the end of the world and it could cause you to over eat more.

No, in fact, you should anticipate giving into your cravings. However instead of cutting out the food that you frequently crave completely from your diet, have it once in a while. Don't binge, but eat in moderation. By doing this you won't feel like you're depriving yourself and you won't have intolerable cravings.

If you're craving your grandmother's pecan pie, but you know that she uses a ton of butter, sugar, and corn syrup, you could find a healthier alternative. There are plenty of recipes online that can offer healthy alternatives to any kind of food. You won't sacrifice a lot of flavor but you will be ditching the empty calories. With a healthier version of that pecan pie, you will still get the pecan pie flavor and texture without the extra sugar.

We discussed earlier that stress and our emotions play heavily on why we over eat and also play into what we crave. It may sound silly, but take a time out and breathe deeply. Instead of reaching for the bag of chips or those cookies, take a hot bath and soak in the tub. The hot water and alone time will allow you to decompress and reflect on the day. This will give you a chance to clear your head. You'll be likely to find that your cravings will subside.

If you find that the bath doesn't help, try and find a distraction. Do you have some chores that need to be done? Go and do them. Go for a walk or jog. By keeping busy, your mind isn't focusing on the craving. People tend to give into their cravings because they could be bored. How many times have you have gone to the fridge because you were bored? I can't count the number of times it's happened to me!

It is possible to trick the brain into thinking that you've eaten something to stop craving something. You could drink some ice cold water.

The cold water jump starts your metabolism so that the water can be warmed up to match your body temperature. This makes you burn calories and gives you some energy. If you are still craving something with a flavor, try a slice of citrus (lemon, lime or orange) to help. This also offers a small sweet taste to help your brain think you ate something sweet. Another mind trick can be to brush your teeth. It may sound strange but think about it. Do you ever brush your teeth and then eat something afterward? That taste alone is to not want to eat anything.

Have you ever noticed that if you're in the mall and you are shopping at the end where the food court is not located, you're fine; but, as you make your way toward the end of the mall where the food court is, you begin craving the food?

The aromas of all the tasty treats can be all too alluring. It's almost criminal if the food court is located at the center of the mall! One option is to avoid going to the mall on an empty stomach. You most likely won't want to eat a cinnamon roll if you're already full.

This is my favorite trick. I take a nap if I have a craving. I find I'm not thinking about eating, and studies also suggest that cravings sneak up on you when you're tired. When you wake up and you find that you are still hungry, you can determine if it is a genuine hunger or if it is still a craving.

You've heard this before thousands of times, exercise is important to any healthy lifestyle. Not only can it help to ease a craving, it has countless benefits. It can improve your stamina, strengthen your muscles, prevents diseases such as high blood pressure and diabetes. And most importantly, it can help you lose weight.

Inactivity is one factor in a person over eating and choosing the bad food that you try so hard to avoid. Researchers have found that when someone exercises and then an hour later see a photo of food, they do not respond the same way as when they did not exercise. The exercise balances the brain and turns off the pleasure seeking switch that yearns for food.

Sources for this section:

http://www.health.com/health/gallery/0,,2034 9566,00.html

http://www.prevention.com/weight-loss/weight-loss-tips/how-stop-food-cravings-and-overeating

http://www.fitday.com/fitness-articles/fitness/weight-loss/7-mental-tricks-to-stop-cravings-now.html

http://www.rd.com/health/healthy-eating/10-ways-to-control-your-cravings/

http://www.healthdiscovery.net/articles/exercis e_importa.htm

What Can I Eat?

Read Your Cravings and Understand What Your Body Needs

Are you craving something salty? Your body is telling you that you are missing chloride.

Chloride is one of the most important electrolytes that your body needs. The electrolyte balances the amount of fluid both inside and outside of your cells. It also maintains your blood pressure and pH balance in your bodily fluids. Your body absorbs chloride in your intestines but your body can be low on chloride due to frequent urination and sweating.

There are a few minerals missing if you are craving sweets. Your body is missing carbon, phosphorus and sulfur. Carbon is found in 18% of your body mass, however it is not pure carbon. it is joined with other compounds to act as a filter for reactant chemicals. It also is an important source of energy for your body.

Phosphorus also helps create energy. It also helps keep your bones and teeth healthy and strong (calcium isn't the only one that is responsible for this task!) It also helps you absorb vitamin B, which helps maintain your emotional state and keep your mind sharp.

Finally, sulfur helps produce collagen, which forms cell structure, artery walls, and connective tissue. It will also help give your hair, skin and nails the strength that ladies look for. Sulfur also helps treat arthritis and some kind of skin disorders. However to sulfur is often used topically in these cases.

If you crave fatty foods, your body is looking for calcium. As we know, calcium is needed to keep our teeth and bones strong. It also is necessary to help our body produce the hormones and enzymes that are used in many of our body's functions.

What Can I Eat to Help These Cravings?

Pretzels are a good snack if you crave salt. For a two ounce package of pretzels you will be consuming 218 calories, whereas if you eat a 2 ounce package of chips you will be eating 307 calories. They both are high in the carb count, but pretzels are lower in fat. Chips are 21 grams of fat and pretzels have only 2 grams of fat.

Nuts and Seeds can be a questionable option, because they are high in calories and fat, but they offer some health benefits, such as omega-3 fatty acids. If eaten in moderation, they can cut the salt craving.

Pickles and olives are salty but they are low in calories. By snacking on just a few pickle slices or a couple of olives, you are getting that salt but none of the other bad fats and high calories.

Cottage cheese can cut the salt cravings while giving you protein and calcium. Want to be even healthier, select the low fat or fat free options and add some fruit for a different taste. What I like to do is cut up some red onion and add some black pepper--it's delicious!

If you're eating a salad and want something salty, grab the balsamic vinaigrette. This dressing is loaded with unsaturated fats, these are good for you. The balsamic vinegar has that salty bite that you're looking for.

Fresh fruits are an excellent source of sweetness. Strawberries, grapes, apples, oranges, pineapple, they are all sweet and offer excellent sources of a variety of vitamins and nutrients that your body already needs.

Would you be surprised to know that eating seafood can help with the sugar cravings? Seafood such as oysters, crab, tuna and salmon have zinc and niacin in them. Zinc and Niacin help release serotonin and this will curb the craving all together.

Since processed foods have high fructose corn syrup, it would be logical that when eating a lot of these foods, we will crave them. By choosing whole grains and unprocessed foods can stop the insulin spikes which encourage those cravings. Try a baked potato with low fat toppings. The potato promotes the release of serotonin.

Dark chocolate can help curb the craving too. While it is candy, it doesn't have as much sugar as a milk chocolate bar does. Plus dark chocolate has antioxidants in it, so that's a plus!

Sources for this section:

http://www.fitday.com/fitness-articles/nutrition/vitamins-minerals/why-do-we-need-phosphorus.html

http://www.klutchclub.com/2012/05/08/what-youre-really-craving/

http://www.livestrong.com/article/441274-how-does-sulfur-help-the-body/

http://ods.od.nih.gov/factsheets/Calcium-QuickFacts/

http://www.womenshealthmag.com/nutrition/satisfy-food-cravings

http://www.webmd.com/diet/features/the-facts-about-food-cravings

Healthier Options

Some Healthier Fast Food Selections

There are times when we just don't want to cook at home, or you're on the road and need something to eat, or you just feel like having a nice evening out. The problem with dining out is most of the food is packed full of the very things you are trying to avoid! Not only that, but the portion sizes are enough to feed a small army.

Here is a compilation of some ideas that you can order that won't put a damper on your weight loss/stopping to over eat.

McDonalds:

- **Premium Grilled Chicken Sandwich (No Mayo)** - 370 calories, 4.5g fat, 1,110mg sodium
- **Premium Asian Salad with Grilled Chicken** - 300 calories, 10g fat, 890mg sodium
- **Fruit and Yogurt Parfait** - 160 calories, 2g fat , 85mg sodium

- **Plain Hamburger** - 250 calories, 9 g of fat and 520 mg of sodium
- **Grilled Honey Mustard Snack Wrap** - 260 calories, 9 g fat, 800 mg sodium

Wendy's:

- **Mandarin Chicken Salad** - 540 calories, 25g fat, 1,260mg sodium
- **Ultimate Chicken Grill** - 320 calories, 7g fat, 950mg sodium
- **Small chili** - 190 calories, 6 g fat, 830 mg sodium
- **Jr. Hamburger** (without cheese) - 220 calories, 8 g of fat and 490 mg of sodium.

Burger King:

- **Tendergrill Chicken Garden Salad** - 300 calories, 16g fat, 1,050mg sodium
- **BK Veggie Burger** - 340 calories, 8g fat, 1,030mg, sodium
- **Whopper Jr. or Hamburger** - 290 calories, 12 g fat and 500 mg of sodium
- **Tendergrill Chicken Garden Salad** - 220 calories, 7 g fat, 1,080 mg sodium

Chick-Fil-A:

- **Chargrilled Chicken Sandwich** - 270 calories, 3g fat, 1,260mg sodium
- **Chargrilled and Fruit Salad** - 290 calories, 8g fat, 760mg sodium

- **Fruit Cup** - 100 calories, 0 g fat, 0 mg sodium

Taco Bell:

- **Fresco Style Ranchero Chicken Soft Taco** - 170 calories, 4g fat, 730mg sodium
- **Fresco Crunchy Taco** - 150 calories, 8g fat, 370mg sodium
- **Spicy Chicken Soft Taco** - 170 calories, 6 g fat, 580 mg sodium
- **Mexican Rice** - 100 calories, 3 g fat, 790 mg sodium
- **Fresco Grilled Steak Soft Taco** - 160 calories, 4.5 g fat, 550 mg sodium

Arby's:

- **Martha's Vineyard Salad** - 466 calories, 23g fat, 996mg sodium
- **Junior Roast Beef** - 270 calories, 9 g fat, 740 mg of sodium
- **Ham & Swiss** - 280 calories, 6 g of fat, but it has 1,120 mg of sodium
- **Roasted Chicken Fillet** - 380 calories, 16 g of fat, and 920 mg of sodium

Subway:

- **6" Oven-Roasted Chicken Breast** - 310 calories, 5g fat, 830mg sodium
- **6" Veggie Delite** - 230 calories, 3g fat, 500mg sodium

- **Chicken tortilla** - 110 calories, 1.5 g fat, 440 mg sodium
- **Fire-roasted tomato orzo** - 130 calories, 1 g fat, 410 mg sodium
- **Soups –** Under 160 calories - Cream of Broccoli, Minestrone, New England Style Clam Chowder, Roasted Chicken Noodle, Spanish Style Chicken with Rice, Tomato Garden Vegetable with Rotini, and Vegetable Beef.

KFC:

- **Honey BBQ Sandwich** - 280 calories, 3.5g fat, 780mg sodium
- **Tender Roast Sandwich** - 300 calories, 4.5g fat, 1,060mg sodium
- **Roasted Caesar Salad** - 250 calories, 8g fat, 1,240 mg sodium
- **Hot Wings** - 70 calories, 5 g fat, 150 mg sodium (each wing)
- **Original Recipe Chicken** - 140 calories, 2 g fat, 510 mg sodium

Applebees's:

- **Steak & Portobello** – 330 calories, 10g fat. 1440mg sodium
- **Cajun Lime Tilapia** – 310 calories, 6g fat, 2160mg sodium
- **Weight Watchers Creamy Parmesan** Chicken – 460 calories, 13g fat, 1380mg sodium
- **Blackened Tilapia** – 410 calories, 15g fat, 1360mg sodium

Red Lobster:

- **Snow/Dungeness Crab Legs** – 140 calories, 2g fat, 330mg sodium
- **Broiled Seafood Platter** – 280 calories, 8g fat, 1,660mg sodium
- **Salmon with Broccoli** – 270 calories, 9g fat, 310mg sodium

PF Chang's:

- **Cantonese Shrimp** – 32 calories, 1.3g fat, 216.4mg sodium (per shrimp)
- **Ahi Crisp** – 300 calories, 14g fat, 520mg sodium
- **Moo Goo Gai Pan** – 310 calories, 9g fat, 2380 sodium
- **Steamed Buddha's Feast** – 260 calories, 4g fat, 300mg sodium

Olive Garden:

- **Venetian Apricot Chicken** - 380 calories, 4 g fat, 1,420 mg sodium
- **Shrimp Primavera** - 730 calories, 12 g fat, 1,620 mg sodium
- **Herb Grilled Salmon** - 590 calories, 26 g fat, 720 mg sodium
- **Shrimp & Asparagus Risotto** - 620 calories, 30 g fat, 2,530 mg sodium

Needless to say that when you're eating out, what may be low in calories and fat doesn't always mean it's good. A lot of fast food places and restaurants use salt. Just be wary of this.

Exploring Various Diets

Fad Diets and Popular Diets; what they are and why they are Popular.

In the tabloids you can be certain to find an article promoting the latest diet a Hollywood starlet swears by. Why look! This Emmy Award winner lost 10 pounds on the Cabbage Soup Diet! Learn this day time drama star lost the baby weight by only eating cottage cheese! It sounds ridiculous doesn't it? Most of the times, it is. These diets appeal to a person's vanity, that desire to look good. What the person doesn't take into consideration are the potential side-effects of said diet. All the person wants are maximum results with minimal effort.

There are five types of diets: diets that focus on a few foods or food groups, detox diets, miracle food diets, fasting or low calorie diets, and diets that sound too good to be true. These sound familiar right? These diets may give you the desired effect, however they don't last. A person cannot live off of one food group or consistently eat only low calorie diets. The body wasn't meant to function that way.

The body needs calories to function. It also needs a great number of nutrients, vitamins, and minerals too. By dieting, you are not getting all these things. A lot of diets restrict what you can eat so much that you may be missing some of the essential nutrients all together. You've probably noticed that some, if not all, of these diets tell you to take a multivitamin.

Fad Diets

You have heard them before; some new diet that claims to be every dieters dream. They may say that being on this new and revolutionary diet will leave you feeling terrific and looking fabulous. Many people flock to this diet and hope that *this* will be the one to change their lives. Little do they know, this *new* and *revolutionary* diet is anything but new and revolutionary—much less an answer to their prayers.

Some popular fad diets you may have heard of or even tried are the cabbage soup diet or the grapefruit diet. These are a types of diets that focus on a few food or food groups. Would you be surprised that they aren't very original or innovative? There are several versions of the cabbage soup diet. The premise to the diet is pretty simple. The selection of food is very limited, but one of the main components is...

You guessed it, cabbage soup. Since this fad diet is so restrictive, you will lose weight quickly. However, since this diet is meant to be done in seven day increments, you'll gain that weight back just as quickly. You may even gain more!

Why? Because while you were restricting yourself so much during that week, the moment you get off the diet, you may go straight for the food higher in calories to compensate for the lack of calories from the week before. For dieters, this particular diet doesn't work because it gets boring. Who really wants to eat cabbage soup day in and day out?

Detox diets are exactly as they sound. They are meant to flush your body of whatever toxins may be lurking about. However, dieticians and nutritionists say this diet is just nonsense because your body has all the necessary organs to handle those toxins. Some of the more extreme aspects of these diets call for procedures such as liver flushes, bodily cleanses, colonics, hormone injections, and more are highly suspect, experts say. One popular detox diet is the Master Cleanse diet.

The singer Beyonce announced she used this diet prior to making the film *Dreamgirls* and she lost a reported 20 pounds. What this diet consists of is lemon juice, maple syrup and water. That's all. You drink this concoction for two weeks and the pounds fly off. Well of course it will! You aren't eating anything!

Supplements, fructose (sugar) water, bitter orange, green tea, apple cider vinegar... These are all reported to be miraculous when it comes to weight loss. It is said that these things, either taken individually or combined will enable you to lose weight. Truth of the matter is, there is no scientific proof to these claims. It's just a gimmick. One thing to be careful of though, is supplements. You don't know what exactly is in the supplements and often times they may not be FDA approved. The ingredients could be dangerous. Not to mention they may react negatively to any medication you are currently taking. So be wary of any diet that tells you to stock up on a number of supplements.

Low calorie diets or diets that require you to fast can be dangerous. Let's take the Master Cleanse diet for example. You are basically starving your body. You can only drink that lemon/syrup drink for the first two weeks and then only eat low calorie foods. Whatever weight you may lose during this diet it will be a combination of fat, water, and muscles. Why? Your body thinks it's starving and so your metabolism is adjusting accordingly, meaning it slows down. Since you aren't getting the carbohydrates or calories your body needs it will begin to use whatever it can to keep you going. This will cause you to feel sluggish and you won't have much energy. So, while you may lose weight, when you gain it back (you will gain it back the moment you go off the diet), it will be fat.

Diets that are too good to be true are just that— too good to be true. Some make claims that you can eat whatever you want and do little to no exercise. Really? That's what got me overweight in the first place! A good rule of thumb is if it sounds too good to be true, it is. Don't even try them.

Still, people insist on fad diets. They make excuses. They don't want to be the largest person in the gym, so they think, "I'll lose a few pounds on my own and then I'll go."

Popular Diets

It is believed that overweight people eat too many carbohydrates. This may be true and it may also be why the *Atkins diet* is so popular.

This diet restricts the intake of carbohydrates and you will lose weight quickly. Since the body works off of carbs, the fewer carbs you eat, the quicker it goes through them and begins to use fat for fuel.

According to Dr. Atkins, when the body uses the excess fat it will return to a normal metabolic routine. When we eat carbohydrates, the body turns those carbs into sugar that is used as a fuel for the body. However when we eat too many carbohydrates, we have an excess of sugar and the body can't use it all so it turns into fat. When we restrict the carbohydrate intake, the body will use these few carbs first and then go to the fat that is stored in the body.

For the first two weeks, you are only allowed to eat 20 grams of carbs a day. Fruits and vegetables are almost non-existent during this time. So that roughly equates to three cups of loosely packed salad or two cups of salad with two-thirds cup of certain cooked vegetables each day. You cannot eat any refined sugar, milk, and white foods (potatoes, white rice, and white flour), so you're basically going to be eating only protein and fats for the first two weeks. This goes against everything you may have been taught regarding the importance of fruit and vegetables. Don't worry, you will be allowed to add fruits and vegetables back into the diet after the initial two week period. This is just to get the ball rolling.

Now while this diet may work for losing weight and gaining good cholesterol, may health experts are concerned about the dieters long term safety.

There is no question that the diet works and a person can maintain a healthy weight, however the experts worry that the diet may promote heart disease. They also show concerns about stroke, cancer, bone loss, and those with preexisting liver and kidney problems. The high amount of protein in this diet may be difficult for these people.

Other concerns lie with the lack of carbohydrates a body is getting. The body needs carbohydrates to function, that is a simple fact.

With the Atkins diet, you are not getting enough carbs and it takes a long time for fat and protein to be converted to usable energy. Fruits, vegetables, and grains convert to glucose much quicker and efficiently.

The *South Beach Diet* is similar to the Atkins diet. The South Beach diet, however, is supposed to be more heart conscious than Atkins. South Beach Diet was created by cardiologist Arthur Agatston and he says that "good" carbohydrates are allowed, just not in the first two weeks of the diet (sound familiar?).

After the two weeks, you will be allowed to eat good fats. Well, what is a good fat? Avocados, nuts, salmon, carrots (yes, carrots are on the no no list during the first two weeks), whole grain pasta are just a few of the foods you can bring back into your diet.

One of the claims of this diet is that you will no longer crave carbohydrates. You won't go hungry, you can still eat and feel full. You will just be eating better foods.

This diet is a healthier version of the Atkins, and it does produce a desired effect. However it causes you to lose a lot of water weight during the first two weeks. The loss of the water will cause your electrolyte count to be thrown off balance and could cause you to feel tired and have no energy.

It is suggested that if you do the South Beach Diet, that you should work with a dietician so that you have well balanced meal plans. The South Beach diet isn't bad per say, but it is still a diet that restricts what can be eaten.

Sources for this section:
http://www.webmd.com/diet/features/worst-diets-ever-diets-that-dont-work
http://www.webmd.com/diet/atkins-diet-what-it-is

http://www.webmd.com/diet/features/why-do-we-keep-falling-for-fad-diets

Meal Ideas

3 Simple and Healthy Breakfasts

Feta and Spinach Scramble	Mini Vegetable Frittatas	Oatmeal Blueberry Pancakes
Ingredients: 3 egg whites 1 large handful of baby spinach leaves 1 1 Italian tomato, chopped (any tomato) 1/4 c. chopped onion 1/4 c crumbled feta cheese salt & pepper	**Ingredients:** 5 eggs 2 Tbsp. low-fat milk 1 cup diced tomato 2 oz. goat cheese, crumbled 2 cups chopped broccoli salt and pepper to taste	**Ingredients:** 1/2 cup oats 1/2 cup fat free egg beaters or egg white equivalent 1/2 cup fresh blueberries 1 tablespoon honey Stevia (optional)

	Directions:	Directions:
to taste Chop onion & tomato		
Directions: Spray pan with oil Put on med heat Start with onions cook till desired Add 3 egg whites Tomato, spinach cook to desired consistency Just before you are ready to take off heat, take 1/2 of feta cheese and	Mix eggs and milk in a bowl. Add crumbled goat cheese and chopped vegetables. Season with salt and pepper. Spoon mixture into muffin tins coated with cooking spray. Baked at 350 degrees for about 15 minutes or until "set" and golden on top. You can refrigerate and	Place mix all ingredients in small bowl and mix only until berries slightly broken Let stand 5- 10 minutes to thicken Divide evenly into 3 pancakes and cook thoroughly before attempting to turn Cook evenly on

throw in pan and melt. Slide out onto a plate garnish with the other 1/of crumbled feta cheese on top salt & pepper to taste.	reheat these in the microwave for a quick breakfast or snack. Microwave on high for approximately 30 seconds. Serve warm. Makes 9 "mini" frittatas.	both sides and cook even golden brown

Lunch Meal Ideas

Taco Soup	Spinach and Pasta Salad	Barbecue Chicken Burgers
Ingredients: 16oz. extra lean ground beef 1 small yellow onion, chopped 1 recipe Taco Seasoning 1 (14.5oz) can no salt added tomato sauce 1 (14.5oz) diced tomatoes with green chilies 1 (14.5oz) dark kidney beans,	**Ingredients:** 8 oz small pasta 8 oz feta cheese, crumbled 16 oz grape tomatoes 4 c baby spinach 2 T capers, drained 1/4 t black pepper 2 T Parmesan cheese, shredded	**Ingredients:** 16oz extra lean ground chicken breast 1 egg white 2 tablespoons chopped parsley 4 green onions 1/4 cup whole-wheat breadcrumbs 2 teaspoons BBQ spice rub 2 tablespoons low-sodium BBQ sauce

drained and rinsed 1 cup frozen or canned corn kernels 1/2 cup chickpeas, drained and rinsed, mashed		2 tablespoons plain low-fat yogurt 2 cups arugula, chopped 4 whole-wheat sandwich thins or buns
Directions: Brown the ground beef and onion in a large saucepan over medium heat. Blot any excess grease with a paper towel, then add the taco seasoning. Cook for one minute, then add the tomato	**Directions:** Cook pasta according to package directions until it is al dente (firm to bite). While the pasta is cooking, place spinach, feta, and capers in a large bowl. Before draining pasta, add 1/4	**Directions:** Place the ground chicken, egg white, breadcrumbs, parsley, green onions, and spices in a mixing bowl. Gently knead to combine. Form into four burgers. Preheat a nonstick skillet

sauce, diced tomatoes, kidney beans, and one cup water. Reduce heat to medium-low, and simmer for 10 minutes. Add the corn and mashed garbanzo beans, and simmer five more minutes.	cup of the pasta cooking liquid to the mixture; toss to combine. Place the tomatoes in the bottom of a colander. Once pasta is cooked, drain it over the tomatoes for a quick blanch. Toss tomatoes and pasta with the spinach mixture.	or cast iron pan. Spray with nonstick cooking spray. Grill burgers 12-14 minutes, turning halfway through cooking, or until the internal temperature reaches 180 degrees Fahrenheit. Combine yogurt with the barbecue sauce, then toss the greens in the sauce. Place a burger on a sandwich thin and top with the greens.

		Makes 4 burgers with 1/2 cup greens per burger.

Dinner Meal Ideas

3 Simple and Healthy Dinners

Cheesy Potato Dish	Honey Garlic Pork Chops	Creamy Parmesan Broiled Tilapia
Ingredients:	*Ingredients:*	*Ingredients:*
2 lb. Bag of Frozen Hash Brown	1/4 + 1/8 cup honey	2 tilapia fillets (5 oz to 6 oz each - if frozen,
½ Cup of Melted Butter or Margarine	3 tbsp soy sauce	be sure to thaw fully before cooking)
1 tsp. of Salt	6 cloves garlic, minced	2 teaspoons light
1 tsp. of Pepper	6 pork loin chops, boneless,	mayonnaise
½ Cup of Chopped Onions	trimmed of excess fat, 4 oz each	2 teaspoons non-fat plain

1 Pint of Sour Cream 2 Cups of Cheddar Cheese 1 Cup of Cream of Mushroom Soup ½ Cup of Milk		yogurt 1/4 cup shredded parmesan cheese 2 to 4 sprigs of fresh dill 1 tsp garlic powder or garlic salt, divided black pepper non-stick cooking spray
Directions: Mix ingredients together in a larger bowl (no particular order to adding ingredients but easier to mix if butter is added last). After all	**Directions:** In a shallow dish, whisk together honey, soy sauce and garlic. Coat chops in mixture. Reserve left over honey mixture	**Directions:** Combine mayo, yogurt, garlic, pepper, and dill in a small bowl. Set oven to broil on high Coat the fish with the mixture and

ingredients have been mixed spray a 9 x 12 pan with Pam and pour ingredients into pan and make even. Then bake at 350° for about 1 hour or until golden brown	for basting. Place chops on greased grill over med high heat, close lid and cook. basting 2 times	place on a cookie sheet that has been sprayed with nonstick spray. Sprinkle fish with the cheese. Place cookie sheet into oven about 6" below the broiler. Broil for 6 to 8 minutes to cook fully. Turn broiler off and leave fish in oven about 5 minutes.

Odds and Ends

Interesting facts you may not know about the food you eat.

1. A 20 ounce bottle of Coca-Cola has more sugar (65grams) than a large Cinnabon (59grams).

2. Starbucks used to use cochineal extract in their drinks to make them red. The extract is made from crushed cochineal beetles and boiled in ammonia.

3. Drying Fruit causes the fruit to lose almost 80% of its nutritional value.

4. By adding lemon juice to your green tea, it will boost the antioxidants up to 13 times than without the lemon.

5. Grass fed beef is healthier for you because it contains 2-to-5 times more omega-3s than cattle fed with grains.

6. In 2011, 29.9 million pounds of antibiotics were sold in the US for meat and production where only 7.7 million pounds were sold to treat sick humans.

7. 62.2% of American adults are overweight or obese. Mississippi is the heaviest at 34.9% obesity rate and Colorado is the slimmest at 20.7%.

8. Egg whites contain more tryptophan than turkey.

9. Cinnamon is an antioxidant that can help lower the chances of getting blood clots, control blood sugar, can improve insulin sensitivity; which all help prevent weight gain and diabetes.

10. People who drink diet soda are 60% more likely to develop type 2 diabetes than those who drink the same amount of regular soda.

11. Aspartame and MSG - chemicals found in a lot of processed foods - are excitotoxins, which cause neurons in the brain to excite themselves to death. These chemicals can promote cancer growth and help it spread.

12. Ever notice why most fast food places have red and yellow somewhere in their design? That's because these colors stimulate hunger.

13. Nutritious food costs 10 times as much as junk food. 19 cents for every dollar you spend goes towards the actual food, the rest goes toward marketing, manufacturing, and packaging.

14. Researchers at Tufts University did a study on restaurant and fast food places to see how accurate their calorie listings were. nearly 20% of the samples had more than 100 calories than what was reported by the establishments.

15. Consumers spend over $100 billion dollars on fast food per year, and that is in America alone.

16. You know that creamy center you love in Twinkies? It isn't cream. It's mostly crisco... The vegetable shortening.

17. Dark Chocolate contain a lot of antioxidants that help the cardiovascular system y lowering blood pressure.

18. The Heart Attack Grill in Las Vegas, Nevada offers free food to anyone who weighs over 350 pounds.

19. Making popcorn is one of the top reasons why people have microwaves.

20. Temperature can affect appetite. If you are cold, you may find that you eat more.

21. Honey is the only food that contains all the substances needed to live. It includes enzymes, vitamins, minerals and water.

22. People who eat organic food are 8 times more likely to die of E.Coli than those who don't.

23. FDA allows frozen strawberries to contain an average mold count of up to 45%.

24. 8 of the most popular food allergies are: milk, eggs, wheat. peanuts, soy, tree nuts, fish, and shellfish.

25. Generally carbohydrates make you feel more sleepy whereas protein leaves you feeling more alert.

26. When you eat junk food, the fats will make you want more food, and the effects can last for several days.

27. The bright orange colors of carrots tell you they're an excellent source of Vitamin A which is important for good eyesight, especially at night. Vitamin A helps your body fight infection, and keeps your skin and hair healthy!

28. Fruited yogurt has twice as much sugar as Lucky Charms. Some greek yogurt has more sugar per ounce than Coca Cola.

29. Foods that claim to be "low sugar" and are "diet" often contain saccharine or aspartame. These have been proven to cause weight gain.

30. The CFC (Children's Food Campaign) has established that some baby contain as much, if not more, saturated fat and sugar as junk food.

Conclusion

Looking back in life I realize how easy it is to succumb to my food cravings. I've always dealt with my emotions with food, and they were never good foods. They were foods that had addictive qualities and I craved them constantly. If you're like me, you've experienced something similar.

You may have struggled with saying no during holiday dinners or parties. You may have stopped at the local fast food place and ordered a meal instead of going home and preparing a healthy dinner. We've all been there.

Within these pages, I hope that you are able to walk away knowing something new; be it why we eat when we are emotional or what foods we can eat that are healthier. It was my intention to relay information that I have learned to you, a fellow over eater.

One of the main things that I hope you remember when you put this down is that food is a necessity. It is in every aspect of our lives; however, it does not have to control our lives. We can break the craving cycle and live a healthier life.

www.ingramcontent.com/pod-product-compliance
Lightning Source LLC
Chambersburg PA
CBHW070943280326
41934CB00009B/1992